WITHDRAWN

manners

last straw strategies

last straw strategies

manners

Michelle Kennedy

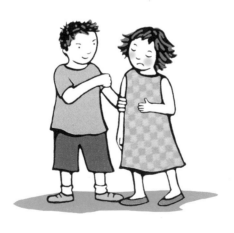

BARRON'S

First edition for the United States, its territories
and possessions, and Canada published in 2004 by
BARRON'S EDUCATIONAL SERIES, INC.
by arrangement with
THE IVY PRESS LIMITED

All inquiries should be addressed to:
Barron's Educational Series, Inc.
250 Wireless Boulevard
Hauppauge, New York 11788
www.barronseduc.com

Every effort has been taken to ensure that all
information in this book is correct. This book is not
intended to replace consultation with your doctor,
surgeon, or other healthcare professional. The author
and publisher disclaim any loss, injury, or damage
incurred as a consequence, directly or indirectly, of
the use and application of the contents of this book.

International Standard Book Number
0-7641-2722-5

Library of Congress Catalog Card No.
2003107787

This book was conceived,
designed, and produced by
THE IVY PRESS LIMITED
The Old Candlemakers
West Street
Lewes
East Sussex BN7 2NZ

Creative Director PETER BRIDGEWATER
Publisher SOPHIE COLLINS
Editorial Director STEVE LUCK
Design Manager TONY SEDDON
Senior Project Editor MANDY GREENFIELD
Designer JANE LANAWAY
Illustrator EMMA BROWNJOHN

Printed in China
9 8 7 6 5 4 3 2 1

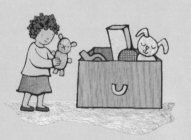

contents

manners
introduction

Manners! It's a little word, really, but it can encompass so many different behaviors. Children have a unique way of often finding the ill-mannered way out and sometimes it seems it is almost impossible to stop them. Whether it's grabbing for food at the table, shouting out a curse word at a most inappropriate time (well, there's never an appropriate time), or hitting, biting, or otherwise injuring a sibling or playmate, there is no end to the number of activities that you as parents must say "No" to. But hearing the word "No" constantly coming out of your mouth can be both monotonous and exhausting. It's important, then, to find other ways to deal with poor behavior. It's also important to determine exactly what is bad manners and what is curiosity, stress, or jealousy—different feelings that can manifest as "bad" behavior in our children. But let's face it, sometimes kids are just ill-behaved because it's either, well, fun, or because it provokes a reaction out of us.

Choosing your battles goes a long way toward easing some of that pain. If you decide ahead of time that being loud, but not mean, is acceptable, then you can take a deep breath when they are loud, and interfere only if things escalate into mean. Prevention is also the key to good behavior in many cases, and the following 99 tips should help you stop bad behavior before it starts—or slow it down when you just can't prevent it!

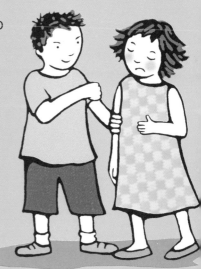

basic
good manners

Sometimes watching your children at the table, especially in the presence of others, is shocking— grabbing for things, yelling at each other, saying, "Gimme!" instead of "Please." When did they become so unruly? But teaching good manners is not as difficult as it might seem. Children are often very receptive to the idea—as long as they are being treated with the same kind of respect—and it's never too early to teach basic good manners. These simple exercises should help both you and your children get on the path to becoming a more polite household.

introductions

Teach your child how to introduce people to each other. Practice some simple role-play at home, then when your child brings home a friend or you go to visit the school, let your child know you expect him to introduce you to his friend or teacher. This simple step to good manners is habit-forming and will become second nature to your child after a while.

basic good manners

the magic words

"Please," "Thank you," and "Excuse me"—use them often! Many times when my children ask me for something— without the required "please"—I'll just stand there, waiting. Sometimes they'll stare back, wondering if there is something wrong with me, but more often than not the light shines from above and they say, "OH . . . please." The more you use them—and expect them—the more your child will understand that they are required. Also, don't give things to your child without that "Please" and "Thank you" attached. It's a small step, to be sure, but an important one.

a thank-you note

3-6 years

Even small children who cannot yet write can send a thank-you note for every gift received. This definitely takes some time on your part as well. Getting your child into the habit of taking time out after a birthday party or other event to sit down and write a note to everyone who gave him a present is not only good manners, but a good writing and creative thinking practice as well. If your child is not yet able to write, or can but likes to draw, let him draw a picture for the giver—perhaps of him using the gift he received.

basic good manners

do a little role-play

Are you taking your children to the theater for the first time? Or perhaps a concert or wedding? Act out the event beforehand—maybe even get dressed up in the fancy clothes you might wear. Running through the possibilities before you go can prevent a lot of issues before they come up. Teach your child how to sit properly (important for girls sometimes) and how to keep her hands in her lap during the "quiet parts." And take some silent activity along for your little one to do in those quiet parts. If she knows what you expect beforehand, she can prepare for it. Letting her know how much you appreciate her efforts (and understand how hard it can be) is very important as well.

talk on the phone

3-6 years

Another great role-play activity is talking on the phone. Even smaller children can be taught how to answer the phone properly, introducing themselves, greeting the respondent, and asking politely to talk with their friend. As children get older they can learn about taking messages or telling people to call back (handy if you're in the bathroom!).

It is important to determine a time when they can accept calls from other children (I've had some boisterous five-year-olds call my house at 10 P.M. when my five-year-old has been long asleep) and make calls themselves.

basic good manners
at other people's houses

I will never forget the day my son had a few friends over and a couple of boys went immediately to the kitchen (without my son) and started pulling things out of the fridge! Now, I will always let my kids eat pretty much what they want when they have friends over, but I thought this was just rude! So I grilled my son and made sure he did not act the

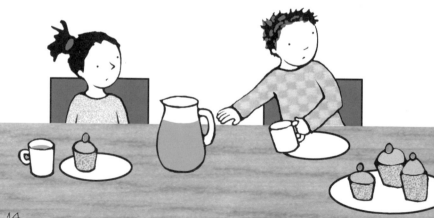

same way at other people's houses. Go over these rules with your children. Let them know that they should eat what they are served and not complain about it, or reply with a polite, "No, thank you." They should also wait until they are offered food or drink, rather than asking for it. If they are really thirsty and are not offered anything, they can ask for a glass of water, not soda or juice. Children who are polite at their friends' houses are welcome guests—for both their friends and their parents!

basic good manners

offering gifts

Teach your child to take along a little token of appreciation when he is invited to someone else's house. A small bunch of wild flowers or a few homemade cookies is enough to show his appreciation. This lesson will last a lifetime so, hopefully, in the distant future, when he goes to his in-laws' house, he will remember to bring a bottle of wine or a nice bouquet for his mother-in-law!

eating together

One of the best ways to ensure good table manners is to eat together for at least one meal a day. Make sure no one begins their meal without everyone being seated, and that no one leaves until everyone is done. It doesn't matter what meal it is—breakfast, lunch, or dinner—but getting the family together for a meal, at least most days, will give your child (even a very young one) an example to strive for and experience in a group setting. If your child always eats by himself in the high chair or in front of the TV, then how will he know how to act in a restaurant or at a large holiday dinner? Remember, if the rules are the same for eating in and eating out, they are much more likely to be followed.

3-6 years **birthday greetings . . .**

At a birthday party, children's writer Jennifer Hartman says, "The birthday child should greet friends and party guests at the door, take their gifts, and show them politely to where the party is taking place. If this is not possible, the birthday child should, at a minimum,

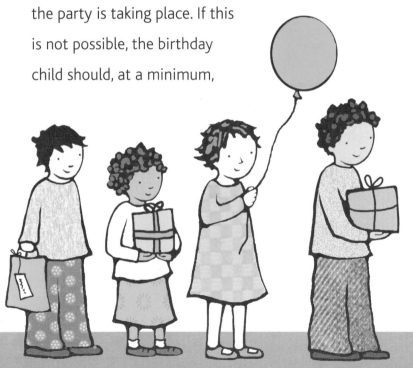

greet each guest at the party area and place the gifts on the gift table." This is important, not only as a lesson in manners, but as a lesson in good friendship. As much as your child is the special one on this day, she needs to realize that going to a party is a big deal for a lot of kids and it's important to make each child feel special.

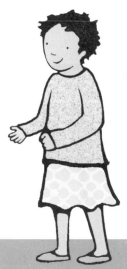

Welcoming a child to the fun and then taking them to the door and saying "Thank you" is a good way for your child to show that she cares about each guest.

basic good manners
. . . and good-byes

By the same token, the birthday child at a party should also be sure to say good-bye and thank you to each of her guests. Teaching your children to take time out, even on a special day, will remind them that even on birthdays, other people's feelings need to be acknowledged. (Sometimes we all need this reminder!) A personal good-bye will make the child who leaves feel special and encourage the birthday girl to think about and acknowledge her friend and the gift she received earlier.

fill in the missing words 3-6 years

Lewena Bayer and Karen Mallett (a.k.a. "The Etiquette Ladies"), who teach classes on manners for children (and adults), say that parents and children can discuss together completing sentences like this: "If there is a new boy in school and he doesn't know anyone, I can show him respect by . . ."; "If I have a whole box of chocolate cookies and my friend doesn't have any, I can show respect by . . . ." Discussing simple issues, like inviting a quiet or shy child to play, goes a long way toward helping a child develop courtesy and kindness.

teaching happy
obedience

This isn't a guide to teaching your child how to blindly follow your every command, because, let's be real, that will never happen. However, what you can do is start thinking of the word "obedience" as meaning behaving with respect for others and yourself. Teaching respect is paramount to raising an "obedient" child, because children who develop compassion and empathy for others will learn how to respect them, and thus behave appropriately. These tips are great ways to get your child, and you, thinking about how your actions affect the world out there.

the king's rules

Get your child to pretend he is a king in charge of the world, and to name three things he would do. Would there have to be rules? What kind of rules? What would happen to people who broke them? You'll find that children are very decisive about such things—then you can apply some of those rules to your everyday life.

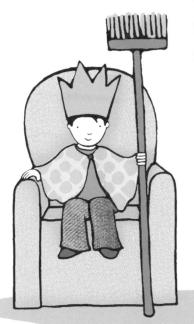

don't turn a deaf ear

"Once," said Kathleen Belanger, a social worker and mom, "I was trying to impress on my children some great truth. They were all standing before me, and I told them, 'The important thing to realize is . . . .' I then thought of something else and said, 'I forgot the bread.' They were listening intently until I put them on hold and turned to something entirely different. I wouldn't think of doing that to a colleague, to someone 'important.' I showed a lack of respect toward

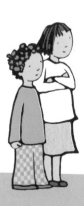

my own children. How can I expect them to respect others? I would like to think that was the only time, but unfortunately I probably can't count the number of times I've turned a deaf ear toward my family." Giving your children the courtesy of your full undivided attention—just as you would another adult—is an important part of teaching them obedience.

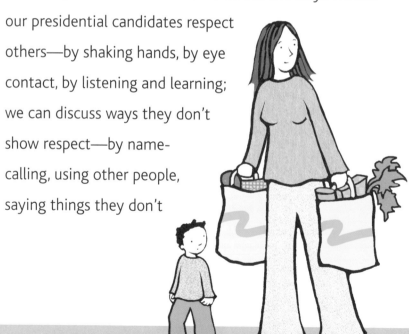

teaching obedience
3-6 years
use words

Belanger also says, "We often assume our children learn things just because they are important, and we forget to talk about those things. We can discuss respect both when we see it, and when we don't. Point out the ways we see our presidential candidates respect others—by shaking hands, by eye contact, by listening and learning; we can discuss ways they don't show respect—by name-calling, using other people, saying things they don't mean. We can use words and actions combined. Try some role-playing to see how it feels."

For instance, if a mom repeatedly asks her kids to pick up their clothes and they ignore her, how does she feel? If a child is ignored by his peers at preschool, how does he feel? If someone thanks you nicely for something, opens the door for you, or picks up something you've dropped, how do you feel? Discussing and using words to describe such actions of disrespect or respect helps to reinforce the importance of behaving kindly.

teaching obedience
3-6 years **let them learn to give**

Have your children gather up old clothes, unused toys, and other items and donate them to a local charity. This is a great way to get everyone involved in showing compassion and respect for others. It's important, I think, that children learn from an early age that it's not all about the getting. This also teaches respect and caring for people outside your immediate circle.

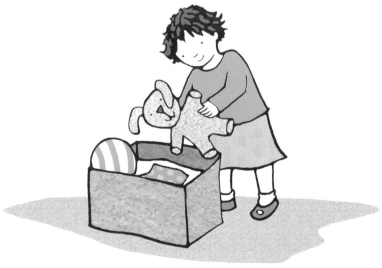

teaching obedience
teach self-respect 3-6 years

Many people who have been hurt over a long period of time lose respect for themselves. In *Teaching Your Children Values*, Richard and Linda Eyre report how one of their children constantly said negative things about himself. Richard decided, one week, to write down all those negative remarks. At the end of the week he reported what he had heard. The boy said that it was terrible that someone should say all those things about another; he would never let anyone talk like that about one of his friends or family members. It was only then that he realized that he himself was the subject. Do your children consent to feeling inferior? Watch *all* the words and actions, even your own. Help each child to see clearly and work constructively, not destructively, to encourage the precious, unique individual that he or she is.

~~teaching obedience~~
3 years and up **discuss compassion**

Identify great examples from history of people who have
been compassionate toward others (e.g., Mother Teresa,
Martin Luther King Jr., Florence Nightingale). Talking about
famous people who exemplified selflessness can encourage
your children to aspire to the highest ideals.

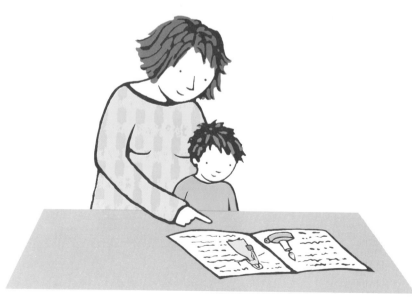

find real-life heroes 3 years and up

Make a list of sports heroes, singers, or actors who do not show humility. Then make a list of sports heroes, singers, or actors who do show humility. Talk with your child about what makes these two groups of people different. Discuss things that the more arrogant folks could do in order to become better role models. Later on, you can remind your child to act a bit more like "so and so" when he isn't being particularly caring toward others, and give him real-life people to look up to and emulate.

promote fessing up

Children are often reluctant to own up. Liam, for example, is famous for claiming that, "Someone else did it," no matter what "it" is. One time I found out that "someone" had put a toy in a new place, and I wanted to reward the child because I thought it was a good idea, but nobody would fess up, thinking I was mad. Finally Liam told me, "Alex did it"—when I knew that it was actually Liam himself. I lavished praise on Alex, telling him how smart he was. Liam couldn't believe it; he came up to me, and said, "No, I did it!" Liam doesn't always come clean now, but he remembers that day and will often confess when he's done something—either good or bad!

encourage self-discipline

3 years and up

Make a list yourself and have your child make a list of three areas in your life that need more self-discipline (e.g., less television, more exercise, less junk food). Discuss them and come up with a plan to change. Hang up the written plan on the refrigerator door. Encourage one another in your attempts to practice self-discipline. This will teach your child that motivation for good behavior can come from within.

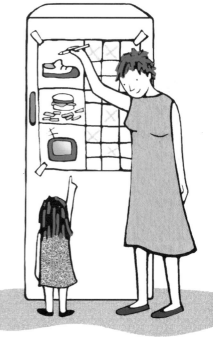

3 years and up **respect possessions**

Children should be taught to respect things as well as people. Show them how to store books properly on shelves. Have them put away toys at the end of the day. Let them help fold laundry and put it away. Also teach them about the proper way to borrow items—and return them. A basic understanding of this type of respect will help your child be more "obedient" when it comes to putting things away or giving things back without them being broken. Kids are often very receptive to the "why" of things. If you say, "Put it away because I said so," they are much less likely to do it than if you say, "Put it away because we don't want it to get dirty out in the yard."

teaching obedience

respect privacy

3 years and up

According to etiquette expert Emily Post, one of the best
ways to teach children to respect a parent's privacy is to
respect theirs. Don't try to involve
yourself in their conversations.
Don't listen in on their telephone
conversations or go through their
belongings. Even when they're
younger, you should knock and
wait for a "Come in" before
entering their room.

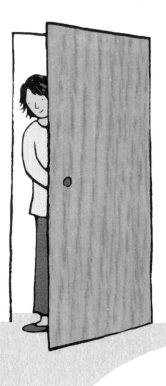

keep that word
zipped!

Oh, it's really funny at first: your precious little two-year-old overhears you when you stub your toe and yell a loud "&%@#$!" and then repeats it in a singsong voice. But it stops becoming cute when that two-year-old becomes a three- or four-year-old who utters that word in front of friends. Soon, it's embarrassing and there is no good way to explain why that word is bad. Why, after all, is the word "chair" okay, but the word "#$%@" a no-no? Whatever the reasoning . . . it definitely needs to stop. But how? If your child starts using inappropriate words in anger, she needs to learn that there are better ways to express her feelings than by calling someone a stupid poopyhead—or worse. These tips, from other parents in the trenches, should help you sort it out.

Keep that word zipped!
"no go" words

3–6 years

Most children under three won't comprehend that certain words are unacceptable. Often, ignoring the offense may be the best defense when dealing with the very young. But after their third birthday they're more likely to understand that some words are naughty. So take action. "Get down on your knees, look your child directly in the eye, and tell her, 'That's a word that we don't use in our family,'" says author Linda Metcalf. To help your child distance herself from such behavior, try to make the words— and not the child herself—seem like the culprit.

keep that word zipped!

time for reflection

If your child persists in using unacceptable language, show him you mean business with disciplinary action. For a four-year-old, that may mean calling a short time-out in a separate part of the room or even taking away a favorite toy. Kids who are a little older may benefit from some time spent in their rooms.

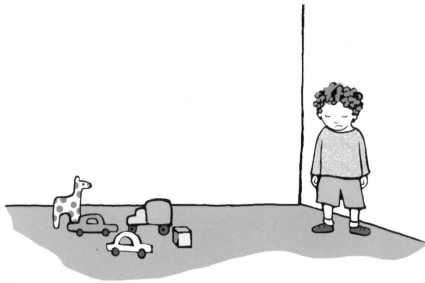

keep that word zipped!
don't slip up yourself 3-6 years

While there are many ways in which parents can help children avoid bad language, there is no substitute for avoiding it yourself. James O'Connor, the author of *Cuss Control*, suggests trying alternative, more acceptable exclamations like "shoot," "blast it," "nuts," "phooey," "for crying out loud," and "dagnabit." Silly terms like "malarkey," "balderdash," and "hogwash" will get your kids to laugh, making them more likely to want to imitate these words rather than bad language.

keep that word zipped!

enlist teacher's help

If your child's outbursts are a problem at school, clue in his teacher to the technique that you're using at home. She may be able to employ it (or some version of it) with your child at school. Consistency between home and school leads to greater reinforcement of the desired behavior.

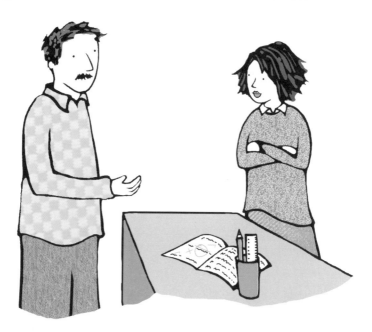

Keep that word zipped!
look for clues

An important step in changing bad manners into good

is figuring out what situations precede your child's

inappropriate behavior. Try to remember what was

happening just before an outburst of bad language, then

discuss it with him after the "offense," so you can pick up

even more clues. Ask him who or what he's angry with—

You? Someone else? Homework? Loss of a privilege?

Himself? Make sure that you intervene as soon as he

calms down after the outburst so that the feelings are

still fresh in his mind.

Keep that word zipped!

establish
calm limits . . .

3-6 years

Often a parent's shocked response actually will encourage a child to repeat foul language. A simple, calm approach works better: "Tom, that is not a word children use. You may say, 'Oh, drat' instead." One mom said, "We convinced him to substitute the more acceptable 'Darn it.' It didn't take long for him to start correcting adults who failed to use this alternative." If the child persists, choose a quiet time to express your feelings, and set specific limits. Discuss why people swear, define what swear words are, and explain why they aren't acceptable in your family. Outline the future consequences of bad language—and follow through the next time it happens.

Keep that word zipped!
. . . and realistic expectations!

How do you act when you're angry? It's hardly fair to expect your child to respond to anger with simple acceptance. Kids are going to get angry. You need to teach, coach, and model the correct ways to respond to those emotions. As long as your child is not using foul language or violent behavior, let him express his feelings out loud.

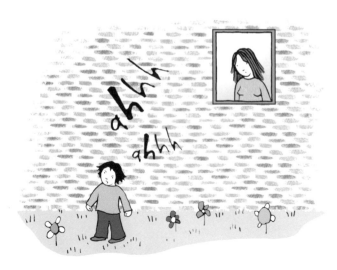

teach acceptable alternatives

Some kids have a hard time understanding their angry feelings. They may believe that they are the only ones who ever feel this way, and that their feelings are wrong or bad. It helps kids when you allow them their angry feelings, even

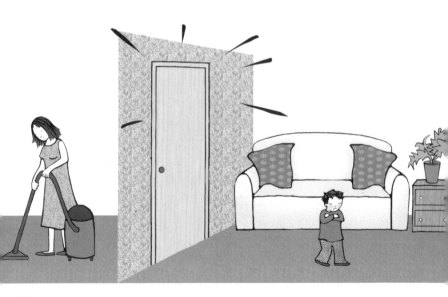

as you set limits on their behavior. As an example, when a kid is crying about a punishment, how many parents respond with, "I'll give you something to cry about"? But the kid already has a good reason to be unhappy! A better response might be, "You're welcome to be angry at me—up in your room with the door closed." If the child then stomps off to his room and slams the door, don't yell at him for doing so! It's a healthy way for him to express his feelings. But when an angry child curses at you, immediately offer an alternative: "That language is unacceptable. You may say, 'I'm so mad at you,' or 'I disagree with you.'"

keep that word zipped!

substitute activities

Teach your child that there are other ways to express frustration, rather than name-calling. Replacement behaviors include punching a pillow, kicking a punching bag, or repeatedly bouncing a ball against an outside wall. Such strenuous activities are safe and appropriate, and help kids express their frustration in a physical way.

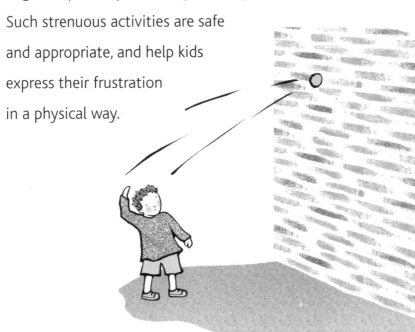

Keep that word zipped!
praise good behavior 3–6 years

When your child responds to her anger in an appropriate way, make sure you acknowledge it (not at the point of anger, but later on!). "I noticed that when you were mad at your brother, you told him how you felt in proper words and went to your room to cool off—that was very mature and responsible!" Or you can take a different tack and encourage "proper" responses before an angry child breaks out. When you see your child getting steamed up, ask her, "What do you want to do right now?" She'll probably be thinking, "Hit my little brother." Giving her suitable alternatives now, such as going outside or to her room to cool off, will give you more of an opportunity to praise her later on.

Keep that word zipped!

why?

Elizabeth Pantley, author of *Kid Cooperation* and *Perfect Parenting*, says the key to stopping children from using bad language is to find out why they are doing it. Reasons include:

- To feel like a grown-up. When kids hear adults swear, it's always in an attention-getting tone of voice. People react. Emotions are on high. The air crackles with static. Older kids try out cuss words to see if they can create the same atmosphere and get the same kind of *imagined respect*. Younger kids are just playing copycat.

- To get attention. Once a child uses a bad word and gets a startled and immediate response from the adults around him, he realizes what a powerful tool bad language can be.

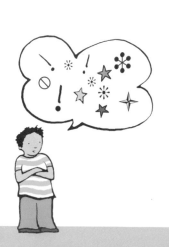 To prove independence. Kids are trying to prove they are separate from you, and that you don't control everything about them. Since you can't possibly control what comes out of their mouths, this is a prime area for rebellion.

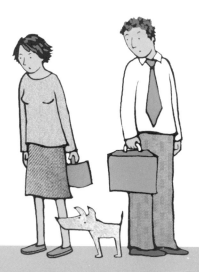 To gain peer acceptance. Often, swearing is seen as "cool," so cursing is just a way to try to fit in with the crowd.

learning to
share

Nothing breaks up a play date faster than a child screaming, "Mine!" All of a sudden, parents are choosing sides and the whole episode can turn out badly. Teaching how to share is a difficult thing. Kids go their whole lives playing with a few favorite toys and then some strange kid comes over and starts messing with them—it can lead to a lot of hard feelings and a lot of confusion on the part of the child at home. But encouraging your children to share successfully is essential, and the following tips should offer a few pointers in that direction.

create a pro-sharing environment

2-6 years

When toys and activities are abundant, children are more apt to share. Toddlers are also more inclined to play side-by-side with the same or similar toys and activities than they are to share any one of them. Puzzles, blocks, building sets, old clothes, hats, shoes, and large pieces of paper for community drawing are all good choices that encourage children to talk and cooperate as they play.

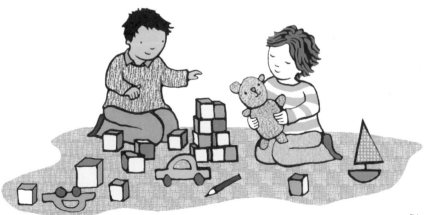

2–6 years

move in closer

Jan Faull, a child and development specialist, suggests: "When your child starts wrangling over a toy, move near the children. Often with an adult in their vicinity, children will stop arguing and decide on their own how to manage the situation, or look to you to help out. If the children can come to a resolution on their own, that's best." By keeping a keen eye on toddlers who are playing together and by staying in close proximity to them, you will encourage children to play nicely, and you will be better able to intervene before conflicts escalate.

get them to trade

2-6 years

When your child refuses to share an object, particularly a toy, you can negotiate a trade: "Carrie needs a turn with the blue doll, so she'll trade you for the pink doll." Or you can set a time limit: "In five minutes Carrie can have a turn with the blue doll." State how long they have to play with their chosen toy, set a kitchen timer or watch alarm, and instruct them to switch the toys when it rings.

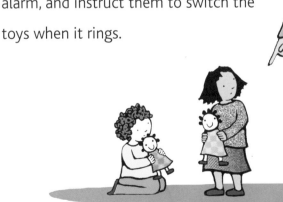

learning to share
don't force sharing on them

2-6 years

Forcing toddlers to share simply models bullying, makes them feel powerless, and may cause them to resent sharing. Adults can help encourage sharing by praising children who demonstrate a willingness to share, by being polite when making a request to share, and by verbalizing the feelings of others when someone won't share with them. Or you can teach your child to ask, "May I play with that toy next?" Rehearsing this technique at home is fairly simple and should make sharing situations easier.

protect their
prized possessions 2-6 years

Usually a child's favorite blanket or stuffed animal provides a
great sense of security. When toddlers are playing together,
don't expect or encourage them to share those special items

with other children. Keep a watchful eye to
ensure other children don't take a child's
prized possession. Explain to them that the
item is very special to that child and that
she does not have to share it. Or put it
away before other children come to play.

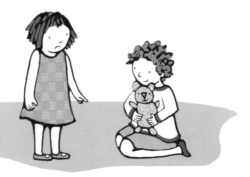

learning to share
have a fashion parade

2-6 years

We have a lot of hand-me-downs in my family, but sometimes it's difficult to get the first owner to put anything into the "handing down" pile. I can't always tell if the older child is genuinely attached to that pair of pants, or just doesn't want the younger sibling to have it! If the clothes will not fit the older child any longer, get her to try on the too-small clothes and give a little fashion show—more often than not, soon she will see for herself that these clothes need to move on.

intervene to resolve conflicts

2-6 years

When sharing battles do break out, intervene—stop the action and take the opportunity to discuss the situation. Letting children fight it out until someone gets hurt, or letting one child get away with taking another child's toy, represents a lost opportunity for teaching them about cooperation, negotiation, and compromise.

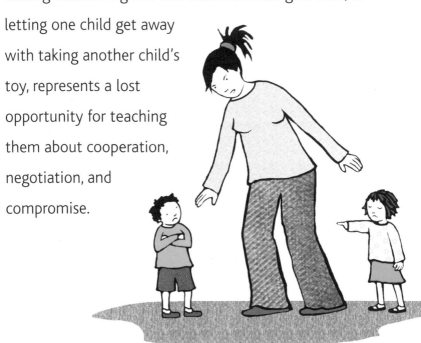

offer toddlers choices

2-6 years

Toddlers and young children like to feel they have some control over their environment. By offering them choices, you are entrusting them with some control, and thus building their self-esteem and helping them learn to make thoughtful decisions. These are character traits that will later serve to encourage sharing and rational thinking.

"one for you, one for me"

2-6 years

A great way to get kids to share snacks is to make a "one for you, one for me" rule. Allow the child to dole out the cookies, but instead of letting him grab a handful for himself, make him place one out for the other child, then one for himself. Doing this deliberately will not only make sure that each child is served equally, but also will remind him to be considerate to the other people around. If it's the dreaded piece-of-cake debate ("Hers is bigger than mine!"), then I do something a little sneaky. If one piece is slightly larger than the other—and he picks that piece for himself—then I give it to the other person. It's a tough one, but it does teach him not to be so greedy and to give the guest the better piece. Don't make the pieces very different in size on purpose, but most kids will notice even the slightest discrepancy.

learning to share

follow through with resolutions

2-6 years

When you are refereeing a sharing conflict among toddlers, be sure to follow through with the "deals" that you help them make. If you told one of the children that he would be able to play with a particular toy after another child had finished with it, make sure that child has an opportunity to do so, even if the toy (or the quarrel) has long been forgotten. Future compromises will be made more easily if the children trust that all parties will cooperate with the agreement that has been reached.

if all else fails,
put it away

2-6 years

If the children refuse to compromise and continue to battle over a particular toy, then play your final hand. Tell

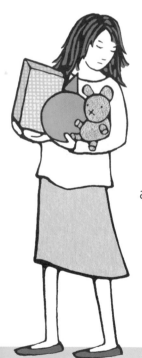

them you will simply put away the toy for another day if they don't play nicely—and do so, if necessary. There will probably be loud protests and tears. Calmly state that there will be no more fighting over that toy today and redirect them to another activity.

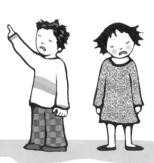

going public

Nothing ruins a shopping trip or visit to a restaurant faster than a wailing child—not just for you, but for others in the venue as well. How can you control your child and still have fun? Do you always have to leave just before the food arrives or before you hit the checkout counter? Not always—but sometimes. These tips can help you prevent awful outbursts before they happen, and give you a way to deal with them when they do, without complete and total embarrassment and your face turning beet red.

set up rules in advance 3-6 years

One mother suggests: "Talk to your child about the shopping trip before you get to the mall so she'll know what to expect once you arrive. You can say something like, 'We're going to the mall, and there will be a toy store there. We can go in today, but we can't buy anything.'" Or before you go into the store, tell her you will not be buying any candy. This way she knows in advance what will be permitted and what won't.

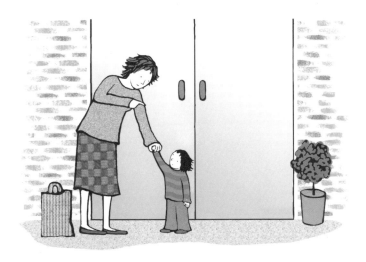

know your child's limits

Some children can be kept interested in what you are doing for a long time, while other children need to move around constantly. Try not to stretch your child's endurance, even if it means cutting short a shopping excursion before you finish all your errands. Remember, children get bored very easily and lose control when they get tired. Don't expect a young child to stay focused while parents debate which bedroom set to buy, or while mom is trying on six new bathing suits. It pays to know your child's limits.

get the child involved

3-6 years

Supermarkets and department stores are a smorgasbord of stimulation: lights, colors, people, music, movement, and things to smell and taste. Have the child choose items off the shelf ("Get me the green can, please") and even try to make it an educational experience by practicing counting, letter recognition, and reading.

3-6 years   **use time-out**

A referee calls "time out" to give players a chance to regroup when they break the rules. Like referees, parents must also use time-outs when their child misbehaves. Examples of time-out include taking the child outside and sitting with him on a bench, turning his chair away from the table at a restaurant, or making him sit on a square tile in the grocery store for a minute or two.

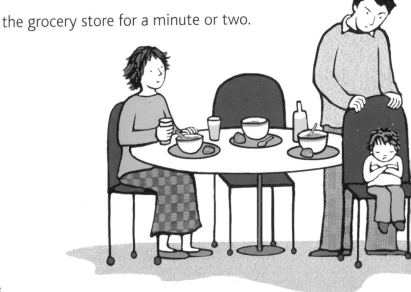

plan ahead

Decide in advance what to do if the child misbehaves—don't just wait for problems to develop. For example, if your child throws a temper tantrum, plan to leave the store with him and wait for the episode to be over before returning to your shopping. You will be able to respond calmly because of your preplanning, and your decisive action will show the youngster that he will receive no "reward" for misbehaving. By the way, temper tantrums are not a sign of bad parenting, and anyone who thinks that a child should be "good" all the time doesn't understand children.

don't reward and don't shout

Parents cannot buy their child's love, and a new toy rarely guarantees good behavior. Too many times parents "reward" misbehavior with a present or the promise of a gift "if you are good in the store." Children who behave best are the ones who get the most praise and attention, not the most gifts. And don't shout—most parents think shouting works, since it startles children and gets their attention. However, the louder and more intensely spoken the instructions, the more likely the child is to disobey. Yelling only adds fuel to an already burning fire!

get away from the scene

3–6 years

What if your child is having a major mall meltdown? "Get the stage lights off the child, and bring the curtain down," advises Kyle Pruett, M.D., clinical professor of child psychiatry at Yale University School of Medicine. "Take her out of the store, even if she's kicking and screaming, and have as little interaction with her as possible until she calms down. Keep chastisement to a minimum —she won't hear you anyway." After the tantrum has ended, you can say something like, "This was hard on both of us. Now let's enjoy ourselves."

going public

assess the situation

You take your kindergartner to a birthday party, and he begins bossing the other kids around. First, ask yourself whether this is typical behavior. If it's uncharacteristic, figure out whether your child is hungry, tired, or sick—conditions that can make him act up. If you've seen this type of behavior before, resist the urge to step in. In this situation, your child's best teacher may be the other party-goers. If you don't intervene right away, he'll learn from the other children that he can't control them. They won't pay any attention to him, and they'll find other kids who will share with them.

tantrum strategy #1

3-6 years

Your little one wants to go to the park; you say no. In front of the entire library checkout line, she screams and hits you. There are two good strategies for defusing the tension. The first is a middle-of-the-road approach: With a firm, you-can't-budge-me voice, tell your child that you're not changing your mind, then take her out of the library. (Or look at the web site *www.babycenter.com*, which offers a range of techniques for coping with tantrums, as well as a host of other baby and toddler topics.)

going public

tantrum strategy #2

A variation is to give her an immediate time-out and some sort of repercussion later. "I would quietly take her out of the library and give her a time-out in the car, telling her that we'll talk about the situation when we're home," says Dr. S. Mark Kopta, author of *Right vs. Wrong: How to Raise a Child With a Conscience.* At home, you can tell her she won't be able to watch television or play for a while.

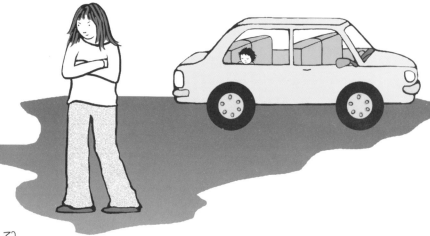

keep her occupied

You're at a restaurant having dinner with some of your extended family. Your preschool daughter is playing with her food—doing what kids that age do when they're bored or need attention. Your relatives look disgusted. The fix: First, tell her firmly that it's time to eat, not play with her food, Dr. Kyle Pruett says. At the same time, engage her in the conversation or give her some activity to do, such as counting the people in the restaurant who are wearing red shirts. You can also bring crayons or a small toy to the restaurant to help keep her busy. The more included your child feels in what's going on at the table, the less likely it is that she'll make a missile out of her meat loaf. If that doesn't work, give her a warning. If the food fiasco still continues, remove her from the room and give her a time-out. As for your family's reaction? Try not to take it to heart.

angry!

Your little angel: She wakes you up sweetly with kisses in the morning, cuddles with you at story time, and lovingly hands you the milk when you're baking cookies. But this same little girl also somehow turns into something resembling your much-dreaded third-grade teacher, complete with yelling and slapping of wrists when she's in a group with other children. Just how did your angel get to be the bully? And how do you stop it? It's always a little disconcerting when you see your own child become the nightmare playmate, but there are some things you can do to make her more acceptable to them. As with anything, the first step is recognizing that it's your child who might have the problem.

learn what calms your child down

3-6 years

Observe how he acts when he's upset. If he usually lashes out physically, or hops on his rocking horse and rides madly, then he's calmed by physical activity. So if he becomes angry while putting together a puzzle, for example, suggest that he runs around in the backyard for a little while instead. Other children may be calmed by more passive activities.

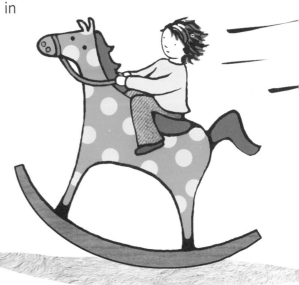

angry!

3-6 years avoid violent influences

Eliminate violent toys, games, TV shows, and movies as much as possible. We had just a little too much "killing talk" among my two youngest boys. I couldn't understand where it came from because I diligently monitor their television watching and video game choices. What I didn't know was that even in some of the video games rated "E" for Everyone, there are still clubs to beat enemies over the head with, and people jumping

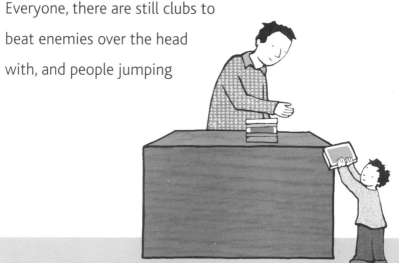

on others until they "die." After a long talk about the
appropriate way to play, and how I wouldn't accept "kill"
as a word to use with each other, I picked out every single
game that involved killing something and had the boys bring
them to a local game store. They received store credit for

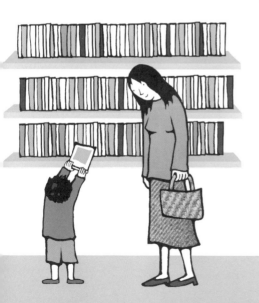

their used games
and, under my
supervision, were
able to pick out
replacement video
games that weren't
nearly as violent.

angry!

watch for biting triggers

3-6 years

Overstimulation is a frequent cause of biting, so follow high-energy activities with quiet play or nap time. A calm, well-rested toddler or preschooler is less likely to use his teeth. And look for triggers. For example, if you notice that your child bares his teeth when a playmate touches his favorite toy, keeping that particular toy out of the play date mix or buying a duplicate toy may stop him in his tracks.

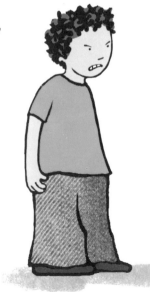

encourage a biter to use words

3-6 years

When a biter starts to bare his teeth, get right down in front of him and ask what he needs. Face-to-face with the problem, he might be able to get his frustrations out in another way. Tell him that when he feels like biting, he needs to come to you and tell you what is going on. Even sounds will work in this case. If your biter is unable to speak very well, encourage him to use sounds like "Aargh!" if he's frustrated. In this case, a yell is far better than a bite. Get him to stop biting first—work on the yelling later, when he can put his frustration into words.

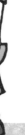

make him
take a break

3-6 years

One mother found this strategy helpful when her son was four: "If he was drawing a picture of his grandmother's dog and couldn't make it look the way he wanted, sometimes all I had to say was, 'You know, you don't have to do it right now.' Knowing that he could stop if he wanted to was often enough to calm him down."

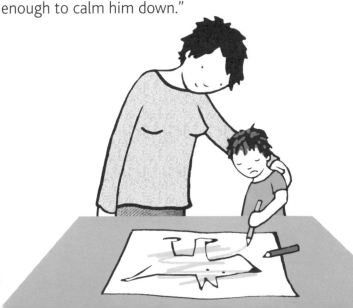

recognize the early warning signs

angry!

3-6 years

Keep track of the things that set your child off on a rampage, whether it's biting, hitting, or screaming. Does she rub her eyes? Clench her fists? Take note and, when you begin to see these signs, intervene with a new activity—or even a nap—before anyone gets hurt. One mom told me that she had her husband videotape her daughter at play (she was about five years old), and then showed the tape to her daughter later on. The mom carefully pointed out the "warning signs" and the bad consequences of her actions, taking care to ask her child what might be a better response when she feels that way. Whether or not you use a videotape, you can halt your child when you see the warning signs and teach her how to recognize them.

3-6 years don't shield your child

The frustration that kids experience in baffling situations can't be eliminated completely—nor would you want it to be, since it is an important part of the learning experience. Experts say that preschoolers need to learn to work through their frustrations. That means slowing down and allowing them time to figure out things on their own. Although you can make certain tasks easier by offering to help out, you should never jump in and take over. Too often, hurried parents complete a task simply because they don't want to spend the time it will take for the child to do it himself. If that happens, set

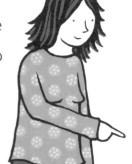

aside another block of time on a day when you don't have to rush, so that your child can practice the necessary skills. A great example is the jigsaw puzzle. Sometimes a child struggles with a piece that is so obvious to you—you are just itching to put it right, but hold back. Ask the child if it would fit better if she turned it different ways. Ask her if she can see a similar-colored piece already in place. Helping her help herself will give her confidence in her own abilities and in the knowledge that you're around to ask questions.

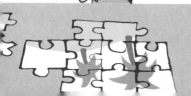

3–6 years   # encourage exercise

To prevent buildups of anger and aggression, encourage your child to do some daily exercise, writes Edward Hallowell, M.D., in *When You Worry About the Child You Love*. Be sure your child gets the opportunity to exercise every day as a way to work off anger and as an outlet for aggressive feelings before they express themselves. Exercise is simply marvelous for the body and brain!

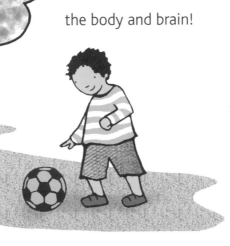

give her space

Help her learn to find enough space for her activity and to give everyone around her enough space too. Sometimes accidents happen and tensions flare when there is simply not enough room in which to play; it may appear to your little one that another child hit her, when in fact that child was bumped by another passing child and was pushed. Young children have a tendency to crowd themselves, and they need to be encouraged to spread out when playing and define their own space.

angry!

reinforce
good behavior

3-6 years

If your child succumbs to bouts of anger, try to catch him being good and then tell him what behaviors please you. Respond to positive efforts with comments such as, "I like the way you come in for dinner without being reminded"; "I appreciate you hanging up your clothes even though you were in a hurry to get out to play"; "I'm glad you shared your snack with your sister"; and "I like the way you're able to think of others." In this way you reinforce good behavior, rather than constantly berating him for getting angry and frustrated.

angry!

stop
the fight

3-6 years

If your child has been hurt or has hurt someone else, you need to stop the fight, say the authors of _What to Expect in the Toddler Years_. Comfort the victim, and offer her another activity. Then discipline the aggressive child, explaining that biting, hitting, and so on are unacceptable. Remind her of the consequences: "If you bite again, you have to sit in the chair for a few minutes." If she bites again, put her in the chair.

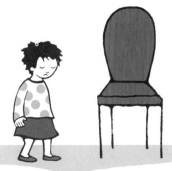

'it's the truth'

"Who broke the vase?" "Not me." "Who poured chocolate milk on the floor?" "Not me." Boy, that "Not me" fella sure gets around. Most children, especially young children, lie out of the fear of being punished. So, how do you make sure your children understand what's true and what's not—and when it matters? And how do you get them to tell the truth—even when they did something bad? That's difficult. But reinforcing that it is always worse to lie goes a long way toward keeping your kids truthful.

"it's the truth"

fantasy vs. reality

3–6 years

Create an outlet for creative writing or storytelling to emphasize the difference between fantasy and reality and demonstrate the proper use of fantasy. This is a good project for an older child who is coming up with some creative whoppers. Recognizing your child's creativity, while emphasizing that report card time is not the moment for a Harry Potter-esque story, can be very helpful. I often say, "Tell me what really happened, and go write that other version down and read it to me after dinner."

"it's the truth"

be proactive about honesty

3-6 years

Tell your child stories from your own life, or read stories like *The Emperor's New Clothes*, *The Boy Who Cried Wolf*, and *Pinocchio*. Offering your child examples of times when you thought it was better to lie—but it wasn't—will let him know that we have all been there and that you have learned it's just better to get the truth out first.

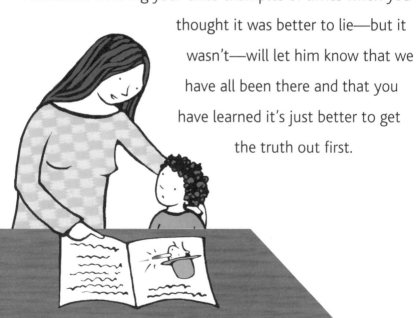

"it's the truth"
avoid telling
white lies yourself

3-6 years

Some parents unknowingly encourage their children to
indulge in white lies for their own convenience. The Practical
Parenting web site (*practicalparenting.org.uk*) presents the
example of Mr. Smith, who was trying to avoid a client by
staying at home and calling in sick. He asked his wife to
call the office for him, and of course his little daughter was
there, quietly observing the whole situation. It got worse
when the telephone rang and Mr. Smith asked his daughter
to answer the phone and say that her daddy was sleeping.
This child would learn that it isn't necessary to be honest
all the time, and that lies can be perfectly harmless.

"it's the truth"

give the benefit of the doubt

When a parent is too rigid or strict, a child may feel pressure to do or say anything to please him. I am often reminded of the episode in L. M. Montgomery's *Anne of Green Gables* in which Anne is accused of stealing a pin. Her guardian will accept no excuse from Anne except a confession. Although Anne eventually confesses, later the pin is found on the guardian's own shawl. "Why did you confess?" her guardian wonders. "You wouldn't listen to the truth" is Anne's reply. Take the time to listen. Bank on your child telling the truth—at least until she proves you wrong.

"it's the truth"
play things by ear

3-6 years

There's no "right" way to act if you find that your child is lying. Your response depends on the nature of the lie and how frequently the lying is happening. "Use your judgment," one mom says. "If it's a toss up, you might decide to let him get away with it. But if the wheels are always 'falling off' his cars, you may need to challenge him." It's a case of matching your response to the situation.

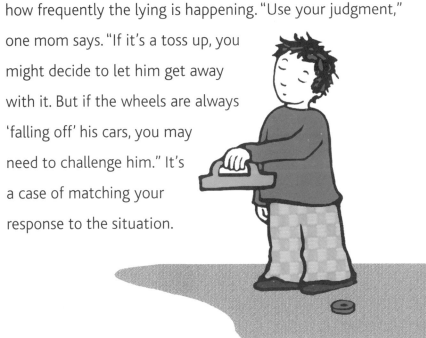

"it's the truth"
encourage him to earn your trust

3-6 years

Privilege and responsibility go together, and when a child lies, the privilege of being believed is taken away—for a time the things he says are suspect and you may even question something that is later found to be true. Being believed is a privilege earned when children are responsible about telling the truth on a regular basis. Not believing your child may seem mean, but he must learn that people who don't tell the truth won't be trusted. Tell your child that you would like to believe him, but you cannot—until he earns that privilege.

"it's the truth"

root out
the cause

3-6 years

If lying is a serious (and constant) problem, try to figure out the cause. Talk to other adults involved in your child's care: Does he seem unhappy? Is he being picked on? Is he seeking attention? Gentle discussion with your child (not in the heat of the moment) may also help you glean hints from him.

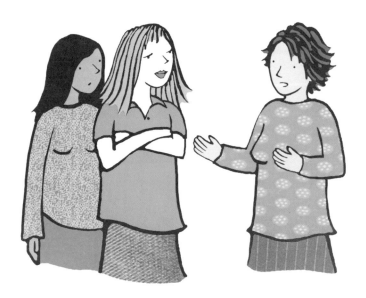

"it's the truth"

stopgap solution

For a short period of time and to encourage an honest response, you can withhold further discipline if your child responds genuinely to correction. "If you can admit it was a lie and that you were wrong, I will not further discipline you for that lie." Sometimes children lie in the heat of the moment, out of fear, and they may immediately recognize their mistake.

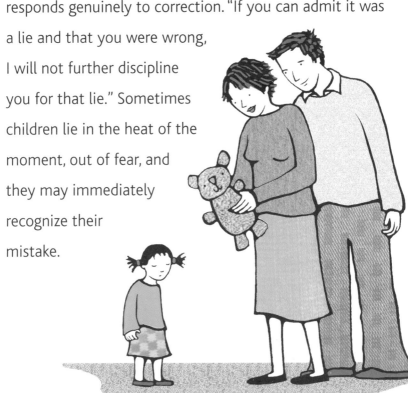

"it's the truth"
avoid muddy water 3-6 years

You may find yourself in a predicament because, although it is impossible to prove, you have a sense that a child is not telling the truth, but you lack concrete evidence. When this is the case, don't push things too far. It's too tricky and you will doubtless have other, clearer opportunities later on to teach the value of telling the truth. Children who repeatedly lie tend to demonstrate it often. Choose the more clear-cut battles and use those situations to discipline the culprit firmly.

"it's the truth"

3–6 years   owning up

Make it easy for your child to own up to "naughty" lies.
Saying, "I see your doll's broken—I wonder what happened?"
will coax the truth more easily than "Naughty girl! Wait till I
tell Daddy." If she does admit the truth, don't be overly angry
or she'll be too scared to come clean next time.

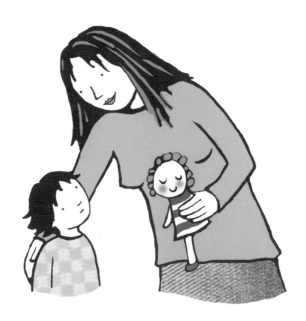

"it's the truth"
cue the truth

Talk with your children about reality and truth, and how
they are different from fantasy, wishes, possibility, pretend,
and make-believe. Dr. Scott Turansky, author of *Eight Secrets
to Highly Effective Parenting*, recommends that children
use cues to identify anything other than reality. Here are
some ideas:

- Possibility: "I think it happened this way . . ."; "I think this
  is the answer . . ."; "I'm not sure . . ."; "Maybe . . ."

- Wish: "I wish this were true . . ."; "I'd like it if . . ."

- Fantasy: "I'd like to tell you a story . . ."; "I can imagine
  what it would be like to . . ."

getting kids
to do chores

It can either be the line in the sand, or it can be the start of something great. Getting a child to do chores is at once a battleground and a delight for every parent who is sick of folding laundry! Most young children start out wanting to help (when often it's easier to do it ourselves) and then, by the time they're old enough to get the job done right, they start avoiding you and rolling their eyes at your every request. Here are some tips on how to get them to chip in.

start early

2 years and up

The best time to start children doing chores is when they are very young—so young that chores are still fun, and so young that they will never be able to remember a time when chores were not just a normal part of life. One mom of three says that a toddler can be taught to pick up a toy and carry it to the toy box as soon as she can walk and hold toys at the same time. At that age, it is a game.

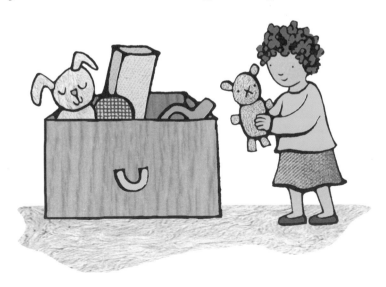

give deadlines . . .

4 years and up

Another mom says, "I have had a bit of success by assigning times for chore completion. My daughter must complete her daily chores by 8 P.M., and not leave them until bedtime, so that I have time to check them. When she has to do something outside of her regular chores and gives me the 'I'll do it later,' I ask her when. I make her assign a time, such as 'I'll start my math homework at 6 P.M.' That way, I can go about my business and just check at 6:01 to be sure she has started. She seems to stick to the times she names."

getting kids to do chores
...and reminders 4 years and up

Another mom comments, "What works best for her now are gentle reminders to set the table, clear and rinse her dishes, put her clothes in the laundry, feed the dog, and other chores that take less than five minutes. When I want her to do something that takes more time, like dusting furniture or brushing the dog, I try to choose a time that's 'convenient,' by which I mean I don't make her put down the latest volume of Harry Potter to brush the dog; I wait until she's already read a chapter or two. Or I may ask her to agree to brush the dog after she's read two chapters, and then I remind her to do it." Trusting your children to meet their responsibilities, and not putting chores above all other activities, should help to ensure their cooperation.

getting kids to do chores

4 years and up **use lists**

Another mom uses Post-It notes on her daughter's door to list three or four things she wants her to do. "She told me she likes the lists, and even crosses each job off when it's done. I have found it helps to make the jobs specific, so it's not so overwhelming. Instead of 'clean up your room,' I write, 'pick up all your dirty clothes and put them in the hamper,' 'vacuum carpet in your room,' or whatever needs doing most. I have even tried lists of homework assignments when she got behind and had so much to do that she didn't know where to start. She helped me write down all the assignments she hadn't finished, and I told her just to start from the top and do one at a time—not to worry about the others until one was done. Once we made the list, she saw that it really wasn't going to take as long as she thought."

getting kids to do chores
and index cards
4 years and up

One mom writes, "What I did with my daughter, who is now ten, is on Saturday mornings, I wrote down all the jobs that needed to get done on index cards or little pieces of paper, one job per card. Then I laid out all the cards on the table and would ask her to pick two. There would usually be around four or five cards with jobs such as 'clean bathroom,' 'vacuum,' 'take out trash,' etc. This way my daughter could see all the work that needed to be done in a more concrete way and was also able to choose her jobs."

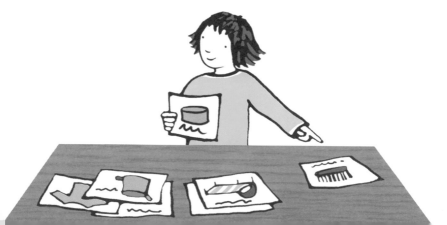

getting kids to do chores

copycat routine

Children love to play at being a grown-up. If they are given an apron, a little mixing bowl, and a spoon when you cook in the kitchen, they will also imitate you when you do other chores. Even the littlest ones should assist you when you clean their room. They can be handed toys to put away, allowed to dust with a feather duster, and help make the bed. Sure, you can do it faster yourself, but you are thinking long-term right now. Parenting for today invariably creates spoiled children. Your long-range plan is to get this child to clean his own room—and as soon as possible.

getting kids to do chores
offer incentives

One mom found that, with preschoolers and older kids, a little parental creativity got the chore done. "I didn't bribe the children," she says, "but I did tell them what we were going to do next and that we couldn't do it if we ran out of time. Story time is more fun than chore time, so I usually had chore time just before story time. The faster we finished, the more stories we had time for."

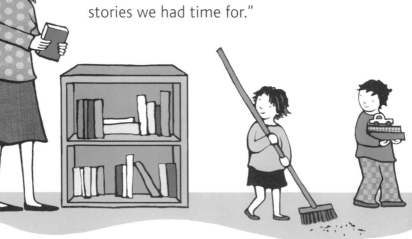

4 years and up

treasure hunt!

Have preschoolers treat picking-up time as a treasure hunt. Get them to pick up only blue things first, or only things with wheels. Ask them to pretend they are robots, or birds, or dogs, and to pick up the way that creature would. Challenge them

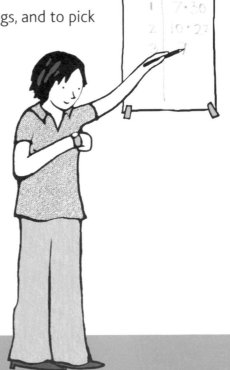

to set a new world record in pick-up. Do this by purchasing a large sturdy basket. Have the kids pick up everything that isn't trash or breakable and throw it into the basket. Time them, then write the time on a wipe-off board or poster with the date. Each time they do it, challenge them to beat their record. Once a week, start over, because eventually they will max out and be unable to go any faster. (Make sure they eventually put away everything in the basket.)

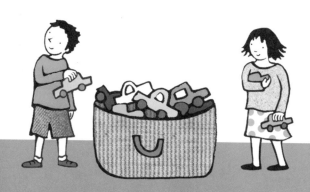

quiz and story time

4 years and up

"My mother always assigned us to work in the same area of the house," one mom says. "While we tackled the living room and dining room, she cleaned the kitchen and fired questions at us. 'What were the names of Columbus' three ships?' 'Who was president when the Korean War started?' 'What books did Laura Ingalls Wilder write?' Sometimes she recited the first line of a poem or famous speech. We had to continue as far as we could and name the author.

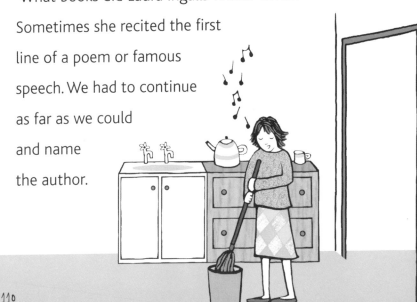

When we were stumped, she gave us the next line and moved on. Other days, we made up what we called talking stories. We each created a character and agreed on a basic plot (when we were working without parents, we were invariably orphans). Then we told the story, each of us contributing as we went along. Favorite stories got repeated with revisions to suit our moods. Sometimes we sang or told jokes we looked up earlier in the day.

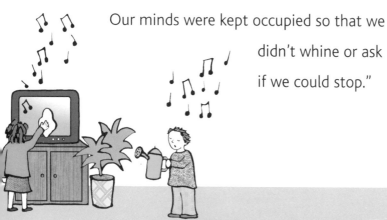

Our minds were kept occupied so that we didn't whine or ask if we could stop."

getting kids to do chores

4 years and up

think big

Don't underestimate what a child can do. Even preschoolers can do their own laundry with help. They like sorting laundry, putting clothes into the dryer, and later folding clothes, as long as you do it with them. That time with you is still precious to them at this age. Make a fuss over their accomplishments, gradually decreasing the fanfare as time goes on. (You don't want them to expect a parade for cleaning their rooms.) Let them participate in all sorts of chores.

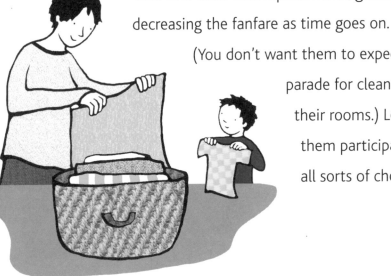

make charts

Older children may need an instruction sheet to help them clean a room without your supervision. The children can go down the list to be sure they don't forget anything, and the itemized chart keeps them from feeling overwhelmed by the number of tasks. Charts may need to be quite specific at first. ("Pick up all the blocks. Pick up all the toy cars. Fold clothes neatly.") Later you can be more general as you discover they no longer need as many details. ("Clean up room. Make bed. Dust.")

when good kids are
bad sports

Think of all the times you let your child beat you at checkers or in a running race across the yard. Now look at the way she rants and raves when someone else beats her. How do you turn your normally well-behaved child into a good sport? It's tough. You want your kids to be competitive and even to win, but at what cost? Teaching a child how to lose gracefully is a difficult, but very necessary skill.

learning from others 3 years and up

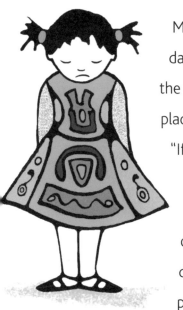

My daughter competes in Irish dancing and was dismayed by the girls who cried when they didn't place. "They're so dramatic," she said. "If I don't win, I just think: 'Crazy judge, what does she know?'" Even though I felt bad for the other parents, I was glad that my daughter had seen an example of poor sportsmanship and could learn from it and at the same time express her own self-confidence.

bad sports

learning what not to do

3 years and up

One mom says that a successful way to foster good sportsmanship is to talk with your children when they are on the receiving end of poor sportsmanship. "My daughters both play team sports and occasionally run up against teams or players who heckle, play dirty, or gloat over a slaughter. We talk about how this makes them feel and how mean it would be to do the same to others. Sometimes the best lessons are learned from being hurt and being on the receiving end of bad sportsmanship." Turn these times into a positive lesson on what *not* to do.

watch your own behavior

3 years and up

Good sportsmanship begins at home. Often, kids who are bad sports feel they are under a lot of pressure from their parents to win at all costs. What kind of an example are you setting? Ask yourself these questions: How do I behave when I'm playing sports or board games with my children? How do I react when they make a mistake? When they lose? How do I behave at my children's soccer, Little League, or football games? Do I ever get visibly angry at the coach or the referee?

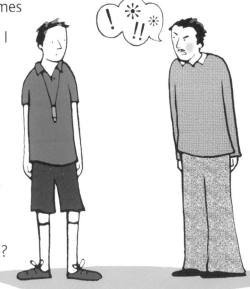

teach by example

If you avoid the issue of winning and losing, a child never learns how to be gracious in victory and defeat. Teach by example: When you win, acknowledge the victory, but never dwell on it. When you lose, congratulate the winner, then say something positive about the experience. With young children, stick to games of chance (like Chutes and Ladders), so that even the littlest player has a good shot at winning.

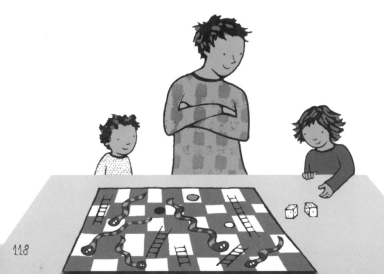

be a role model

Offer praise and encouraging words for all athletes, including your child's opponents. Never openly berate, tease, or demean any child athlete, coach, or referee while attending a sporting event, and refrain from criticizing or condemning athletes' performances when you watch them on TV with your child. During the Olympics, what messages are you sending your child if you honor only athletes from the United States, while rooting against athletes from all other countries? Let your child see you enjoying the sports and athletic activities that you watch and play, and demonstrating that you don't always need to win or be the best to enjoy playing sports.

hidden agenda?

Be honest about why you want your child to play organized sports. What do you want him to gain from the experience? Are your intentions based on providing him with pleasurable, social activities that develop a better sense of self-worth, skills, and sportsmanship? Or do you harbor dreams of him turning his topspin forehand into a collegiate scholarship, or riches and fame? A child's participation in sports should not be driven by a parent's desire to use his accomplishments for other purposes.

you set the rules

It's ultimately your responsibility to teach your children good sportsmanship, both as a participant and as a spectator. If you observe your child engaged in poor sportsmanship—regardless of whether or not her coach corrects her—you must discuss your child's misbehavior and insensitivity with her after the game is over. If a coach is ignoring, allowing, or even encouraging poor sportsmanship, you need to make your objections known to the coach in a private discussion afterward.

bad sports

watching and learning

3 years and up

Whether you're watching sports on TV or attending a high school event, you can always find "teachable moments." Ask your child her opinions of: players who taunt their opponents; the costs to the team of a technical foul, or being ejected for unsportsmanlike conduct; and the appropriate behavior of opposing players toward one another after a game. Ask open-ended questions and listen more than you talk or lecture.

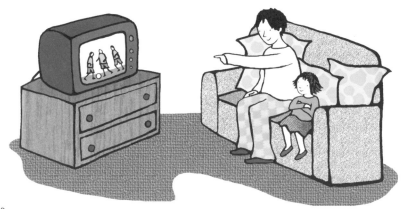

offer some encouragement

"I try to congratulate my daughter a lot," one mom writes, "but also say things like 'Okay, you missed, just try again,' so she doesn't think things always go her way. I also try to be a good sport with my husband. I'll tell him, 'Nice throw,' and he usually does the same! I think our daughter will pick up that playing together is fun, and not about winning." And another mom says, "I tell my four-year-old son and two-year-old daughter, who are constantly racing each other, that they will always be a winner as long as they finish (eating, running, or whatever the race may be)."

bad sports

3 years and up

literary advice

"I read Dr. Seuss's *Oh, the Places You'll Go!* often to Matt, my four-year-old," one mom says. "The book isn't specifically about competition, but talks about the highs and lows of our journey through life, and how you'll succeed—except when you don't. It's a fun way to reinforce the idea that no one can win all the time."

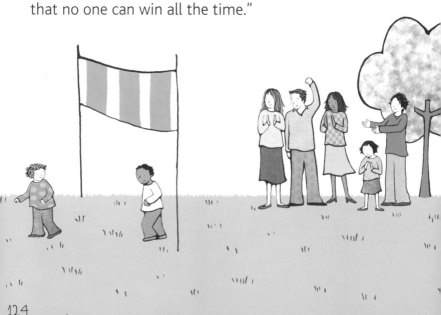

equal praise

Another mom had trouble convincing her children that winning wasn't important. "I think it's a losing battle to try and convince kids that winning isn't important—kids believe it's important and they want to win, no matter what you say. My four-year-old, Julian, has just started to figure out that he likes to win and he hates to lose. So even when he doesn't win—like if he's racing with a bunch of his friends and comes in dead last—he'll still announce, 'I win!' Instead of pointing out to him, 'No, you didn't win,' I try to shift the focus from winning and losing by saying, 'Oh, you are *all* really fast!'"

further reading

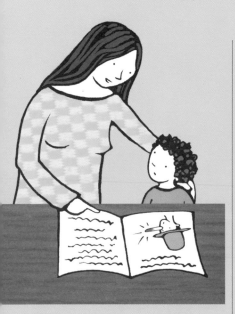

ARLENE EISENBERG, HEIDI E. MURKOFF, AND SANDEE E. HATHAWAY
What to Expect in the Toddler Years.
New York: Workman Publishing, 1994.

RICHARD AND LINDA EYRE.
Teaching Your Children Values.
New York: Fireside, 1993.

EDWARD HALLOWELL, M.D.
When You Worry About the Child You Love.
New York: Simon & Schuster, 1996.

MARK KOPTA.
Right vs Wrong: How to Raise a Child with a Conscience.
Bloomington, IN: Indiana University Press, 2000.

LINDA METCALF.
Parenting Toward Solutions.
Englewood Cliffs, NJ: Prentice Hall, 1996.

JAMES O'CONNOR.
Cuss Control.
New York: Three Rivers Press, 2000.

ELIZABETH PANTLEY.
Kid Cooperation
Oakland, CA: New Harbinger, 1996.

ELIZABETH PANTLEY.
Perfect Parenting.
New York: McGraw-Hill, 1998.

DR. SEUSS.
Oh, the Places You'll Go!
New York: Random House, 1990.

DR. SCOTT TURANSKY.
Eight Secrets to Highly Effective Parenting.
Lawrenceville, NJ: Effective Parenting, 1996.

USEFUL WEB SITES
www.babycenter.com
www.practicalparenting.org.uk

notes

Acknowledgments

I would like to thank my children, my husband John Hogan, my mother, and Rebecca Saraceno and Mandy Greenfield for all their help and encouragement.

index